COLLAGEN DIET COOKBOOK

Delicious Recipes to Glow Your Skin, strengthen joints and a younger you.

Sophia Lawson

Copyright

TABLE OF CONTENTS

Introduction

Unlocking Your Body's Natural Beauty and Strength

Have you heard the whispers of a hidden hero in the realm of health and wellness? A whisper fueled by glowing skin, supple joints, and a newfound vibrancy? That, my friend, is the murmur of the collagen revolution, and you're invited to join the movement.

This chapter is your gateway to unlocking the secrets of this powerful protein, collagen. But before we dive into the science and scrumptious recipes, let's take a moment to understand why collagen has become the newest darling of the wellness world.

What is Collagen? The Building Block of You:

Collagen, simply put, is the glue that holds you together. It's the most abundant protein in your body, forming the scaffolding for your skin, bones, joints, muscles, and even your gut lining. Think of it as the invisible architect, silently responsible for your youthful bounce, smooth complexion, and pain-free movement.

But time, unfortunately, throws a wrench in these well-oiled works. As we age, our collagen production naturally declines, leading to the unwelcome whispers of wrinkles, creaky joints, and achy muscles. This is where the collagen revolution steps in, offering a delicious and empowering way to fight back.

Why a Collagen Diet? More Than Just a Buzzword:

The collagen diet isn't about trendy restrictions or unsustainable fads. It's about embracing a conscious approach to nourishing your body with the very protein it needs to thrive. By incorporating collagen-rich foods and recipes into your daily life, you're not just chasing trends, you're investing in your long-term health and well-being.

So, what exactly are the benefits? Consider this:

- Radiant Skin: Collagen is the secret weapon of youthful skin, boosting elasticity and minimizing the appearance of wrinkles. Imagine a plump, dewy complexion that glows from within – that's the collagen diet promise.

- Joint Support: Collagen lubricates and strengthens your joints, offering relief from pain and stiffness. No more wincing with every step; the collagen revolution paves the way for pain-free movement.
- Gut Health Hero: Collagen supports your gut lining, promoting healthy digestion and a balanced microbiome. Say goodbye to bloating and discomfort, and hello to a happy, well-functioning gut.
- Muscle Mender: Collagen repairs and rebuilds muscle tissue, helping you recover faster from workouts and maintain lean muscle mass. Get ready to conquer your fitness goals with the power of collagen on your side.
- Total Wellness: From promoting strong hair and nails to boosting energy levels and cognitive function, the benefits of collagen extend far beyond the surface. Think of it as a holistic approach to well-being, nourishing your body from the inside out.

Unlocking the Secrets of This Cookbook:

This cookbook is your culinary compass on the collagen journey. Inside, you'll find a treasure trove of mouthwatering recipes, from collagen-infused smoothies and savory breakfasts to delightful dinners and satisfying snacks. We've taken the guesswork out of cooking with collagen, offering easy-to-follow instructions and ingredient variations to suit every taste and dietary preference.

But this book is more than just a recipe collection. It's a guide to navigating the collagen lifestyle. We'll shed light on choosing the right type of collagen, incorporating it into your daily routine, and even offer tips on maximizing its benefits through complementary lifestyle choices.

Your Journey Begins Now:

So, are you ready to join the collagen revolution? Turn the page, explore the delicious recipes, and embark on a journey to unlock your body's natural beauty and strength. Remember, your well-being is a delicious adventure waiting to be savored, and collagen is the secret ingredient to a healthier, happier you.

Let's begin!

Collagen-Rich Breakfasts

Fuel your morning with these delectable and collagen-packed breakfasts! Each recipe features the power of collagen, providing essential protein and setting the stage for a vibrant and healthy day.

1. Tropical Collagen Smoothie Bowl with Granola:

- Ingredients:
    1. 1 scoop unflavored collagen powder
    2. 1 cup frozen mango chunks
    3. 1/2 cup pineapple chunks
    4. 1/2 cup plain Greek yogurt
    5. 1/4 cup unsweetened almond milk
    6. 1/4 cup shredded coconut
    7. 1/4 cup granola
    8. Tropical fruit slices (optional)
- Preparation:
    1. Blend collagen powder, mango, pineapple, yogurt, and almond milk until smooth and creamy.
    2. Pour into a bowl, and top with granola, shredded coconut, and your favorite tropical fruit slices.
    3. Dive in and embrace the island vibes!

2. Creamy Collagen Coffee with MCT Oil and Spices:

- Ingredients:
    1. 1 scoop unflavored collagen powder
    2. 1 cup freshly brewed coffee
    3. 1 tablespoon full-fat coconut milk
    4. 1 teaspoon MCT oil (optional)
    5. 1/4 teaspoon ground cinnamon
    6. Pinch of nutmeg
- Preparation:
    1. Heat coffee in a saucepan over low heat. Whisk in collagen powder until dissolved.
    2. Stir in coconut milk, MCT oil (if using), cinnamon, and nutmeg.
    3. Pour into your favorite mug, foam it up with a handheld milk frother (optional), and enjoy a warm, spiced collagen boost.

3. Savory Collagen Scrambled Eggs with Spinach and Tomatoes:

- Ingredients:
    1. 2 eggs
    2. 1 scoop beef or chicken collagen peptides

3. 1/2 tablespoon butter
        4. 1/2 cup chopped spinach
        5. 1/4 cup chopped cherry tomatoes
        6. Salt and pepper to taste
- Preparation:
        1. Whisk eggs and collagen powder together in a bowl. Season with salt and pepper.
        2. Melt butter in a skillet over medium heat. Pour in egg mixture and cook, stirring occasionally, until scrambled to your desired consistency.
        3. Fold in spinach and tomatoes, cook for another minute until wilted.
        4. Serve with crusty toast and avocado slices for a complete and nourishing breakfast.

4. Protein Pancakes with Collagen and Berries:

- Ingredients:
        1. 1/2 cup whole wheat flour
        2. 1/2 cup rolled oats
        3. 1 scoop vanilla collagen powder
        4. 1 tablespoon baking powder
        5. 1/2 teaspoon cinnamon
        6. 1/4 teaspoon salt
        7. 1 cup unsweetened almond milk

8. 1 egg
9. 1/4 cup chopped berries
10. Maple syrup (optional)

- Preparation:
    1. Whisk dry ingredients (flour, oats, collagen powder, baking powder, cinnamon, and salt) in a bowl.
    2. In a separate bowl, whisk together almond milk, egg, and chopped berries.
    3. Add wet ingredients to dry ingredients and mix until just combined. Do not overmix.
    4. Heat a lightly greased griddle over medium heat. Pour batter into desired size and cook for 2-3 minutes per side or until golden brown.
    5. Serve with a drizzle of maple syrup (optional) and additional berries.

5. Collagen Chia Seed Pudding with Coconut Milk and Fruits:

- Ingredients:
    1. 1/4 cup chia seeds
    2. 1 scoop vanilla collagen powder
    3. 1 cup unsweetened coconut milk
    4. 1/4 teaspoon vanilla extract

5. 1/4 cup chopped mixed nuts

6. 1/4 cup chopped fresh fruit (mango, berries, etc.)

- Preparation:

    1. In a jar or bowl, combine chia seeds, collagen powder, coconut milk, and vanilla extract. Stir well and let sit for at least 5 minutes, or until thickened.

    2. Refrigerate overnight for the best texture.

    3. In the morning, top with chopped nuts and fresh fruit. Enjoy a refreshing and nourishing breakfast on the go!

6. Collagen-Boosted Overnight Oats with Apple and Cinnamon:

- Ingredients:

    1. 1/2 cup rolled oats

    2. 1/4 cup chia seeds

    3. 1 scoop unflavored collagen powder

    4. 1 cup unsweetened almond milk

    5. 1/2 apple, chopped

    6. 1/4 teaspoon ground cinnamon

    7. Pinch of nutmeg

8. Honey or maple syrup to taste (optional)

- Preparation:
    1. Combine oats, chia seeds, collagen powder, almond milk, apple, cinnamon, and nutmeg in a jar or container. Stir well and refrigerate overnight.
    2. In the morning, give it a good stir and enjoy cold or warm it up in the microwave. Drizzle with honey or maple syrup if desired.

7. Tropical Smoothie Bowl with Collagen and Granola:

- Ingredients:
    1. 1 scoop vanilla collagen powder
    2. 1/2 cup frozen mango chunks
    3. 1/4 cup frozen pineapple chunks
    4. 1/4 cup frozen papaya chunks
    5. 1/2 banana, frozen
    6. 1/4 cup unsweetened coconut milk
    7. 1/4 cup plain Greek yogurt
    8. Granola
    9. Sliced almonds
    10. Coconut flakes
- Preparation:

1. Blend all ingredients except granola, almonds, and coconut flakes until smooth and creamy.
2. Pour into a bowl and top with your favorite granola, sliced almonds, and coconut flakes.

8. Savory Collagen Scrambled Eggs with Smoked Salmon and Avocado:

- Ingredients:
    1. 2 eggs
    2. 1 scoop chicken or fish collagen peptides
    3. 1 tablespoon butter
    4. 2 slices smoked salmon, chopped
    5. 1/4 avocado, sliced
    6. Salt and pepper to taste
    7. Fresh dill, chopped (optional)
- Preparation:
    1. Whisk eggs and collagen powder together in a bowl. Season with salt and pepper.
    2. Melt butter in a skillet over medium heat. Pour in egg mixture and cook, stirring occasionally, until scrambled to your desired consistency.

3. Fold in smoked salmon and avocado slices. Cook for another minute until warmed through.

4. Serve with toast or a bagel and garnish with fresh dill if desired.

9. Collagen Power Pancakes with Berries and Greek Yogurt:

- Ingredients:
    1. 1/2 cup whole wheat flour
    2. 1/4 cup rolled oats
    3. 1 scoop vanilla collagen powder
    4. 1 tablespoon baking powder
    5. 1/4 teaspoon salt
    6. 1 cup unsweetened almond milk
    7. 1 egg
    8. 1/4 cup mixed berries
    9. Plain Greek yogurt
    10. Honey or maple syrup (optional)
- Preparation:
    1. Whisk dry ingredients (flour, oats, collagen powder, baking powder, and salt) in a bowl.
    2. In a separate bowl, whisk together almond milk, egg, and berries.

3. Add wet ingredients to dry ingredients and mix until just combined. Do not overmix.
4. Heat a lightly greased griddle over medium heat. Pour batter into desired size and cook for 2-3 minutes per side or until golden brown.
5. Serve with a dollop of plain Greek yogurt and a drizzle of honey or maple syrup if desired.

10. Collagen Chia Seed Pudding with Mango and Coconut Milk:

- Ingredients:
    1. 1/4 cup chia seeds
    2. 1 scoop vanilla collagen powder
    3. 1 cup unsweetened coconut milk
    4. 1/4 teaspoon vanilla extract
    5. 1/2 mango, chopped
    6. Coconut flakes
- Preparation:
    1. In a jar or bowl, combine chia seeds, collagen powder, coconut milk, and vanilla extract. Stir well and let sit for at least 5 minutes, or until thickened.

2. Refrigerate overnight for the best texture.
3. In the morning, top with chopped mango and coconut flakes. Enjoy a refreshing and collagen-packed breakfast!

Lunchtime Delights

Hungry for lunch but craving something delicious and collagen-packed? Look no further! Here are 5 more stunning recipes to fuel your afternoon with protein and vibrant flavors:

1. Collagen-Infused Chicken Caesar Salad with Avocado and Parmesan (Serves 1):

- Ingredients:
    1. Grilled or baked chicken breast, sliced
    2. Romaine lettuce
    3. Croutons
    4. Avocado slices
    5. Parmesan cheese
    6. Caesar dressing with 1 scoop of unflavored collagen powder mixed in
- Preparation:
    1. Toss romaine lettuce with Caesar dressing and collagen mix.
    2. Top with sliced chicken, avocado, croutons, and Parmesan cheese.
    3. Enjoy a classic Caesar with a collagen twist!

2. Rainbow Veggie and Hummus Wrap with Collagen-Spiced Tofu (Serves 1):

- Ingredients:
    1. Whole wheat tortilla or pita bread
    2. Hummus with 1 scoop of unflavored collagen powder mixed in
    3. Mixed greens
    4. Shredded carrots, cucumber, bell peppers, and any other veggie you love
    5. Crumbled spiced tofu (pan-fry or bake tofu with your favorite spices like cumin, coriander, and turmeric)
- Preparation:
    1. Spread hummus on your tortilla or pita bread.
    2. Layer on greens and veggies. Top with crumbled spiced tofu.
    3. Roll it up and enjoy a colorful and protein-packed lunch!

3. Collagen-Boosted Lentil Soup with Roasted Vegetables and Whole Wheat Bread (Serves 2):

- Ingredients:
    1. 1 tablespoon olive oil
    2. 1 onion, chopped

3. 2 cloves garlic, minced
4. 1 cup lentils, rinsed
5. 4 cups vegetable broth
6. 1 scoop vegetable collagen peptides
7. Diced carrots, potatoes, and celery
8. Fresh herbs (thyme, rosemary, etc.)
9. Salt and pepper to taste
10. Whole wheat bread for dipping

- Preparation:
    1. Sauté onion and garlic in olive oil until softened. Add lentils, broth, collagen peptides, veggies, and herbs. Simmer for 30 minutes, or until lentils are tender.
    2. Serve warm with a slice of whole wheat bread for a comforting and collagen-rich lunch.

4. Tropical Tuna Salad Sandwich with Collagen Yogurt Sauce and Sprouts (Serves 1):

- Ingredients:
    1. Tuna salad (canned tuna mixed with mayonnaise, celery, red onion, and dill) with 1 scoop of unflavored collagen powder mixed in
    2. Whole wheat bread
    3. Mixed greens

4. Tomato slices
5. Collagen yogurt sauce (mix plain Greek yogurt with 1 scoop of unflavored collagen powder, lemon juice, and dill)
6. Sprouts

- Preparation:
    1. Spread collagen tuna salad on your bread.
    2. Layer on greens, tomato slices, and sprouts.
    3. Drizzle with collagen yogurt sauce and enjoy a refreshing and flavorful lunch!

5. Spicy Black Bean and Quinoa Salad with Collagen Avocado Dressing (Serves 2):

- Ingredients:
    1. 1 cup cooked quinoa
    2. 1 (15-oz) can black beans, rinsed and drained
    3. 1 corn cob, kernels removed
    4. Chopped red onion, bell peppers, and cilantro
    5. Lime juice, olive oil, cumin, chili powder, and salt to taste

6. Collagen avocado dressing (blend avocado with 1 scoop of unflavored collagen powder, lime juice, cilantro, and spices)

- Preparation:
    1. Combine quinoa, black beans, corn, and veggies in a bowl.
    2. Whisk together lime juice, olive oil, spices, and collagen avocado dressing.
    3. Pour dressing over the salad and toss to coat. Enjoy a vibrant and collagen-rich salad fiesta!

6. Rainbow Veggie Wrap with Collagen-Marinated Tofu (Serves 1):

- Ingredients:
    - 1/2 block extra-firm tofu, sliced and marinated in 1 tablespoon collagen peptides, soy sauce, and your favorite spices (try ginger, garlic, sesame oil)
    - Whole wheat tortilla or pita bread
    - Baby spinach
    - Shredded carrots, bell peppers, cucumber, and any other veggie you love

- o Hummus or tahini sauce
  - o Fresh herbs (cilantro, mint, etc.)
- Preparation:
  1. Pan-fry or bake your marinated tofu until golden brown and crispy.
  2. Warm your tortilla or pita bread. Spread hummus or tahini sauce on one side.
  3. Layer on spinach, veggies, tofu, and fresh herbs. Roll it up and enjoy a burst of color and collagen-rich goodness!

7. Collagen-Spiced Quinoa Bowl with Roasted Butternut Squash and Chickpeas (Serves 2):

- Ingredients:
  1. 1 cup quinoa, cooked according to package instructions
  2. 1 scoop vegetable collagen powder
  3. 1 butternut squash, diced and roasted with olive oil, rosemary, and salt
  4. 1 can chickpeas, drained and rinsed
  5. Your favorite leafy greens
  6. Lemon tahini dressing (mix lemon juice, tahini, water, and spices)
- Preparation:

1. Toss cooked quinoa with collagen
2. Assemble your bowls with quinoa, roasted butternut squash, chickpeas, and greens, and drizzle with lemon tahini dressing. A satisfying medley of flavors and textures!

8. Salmon Salad with Collagen Yogurt Dressing and Crispy Kale Chips (Serves 1):

- Ingredients:
    - 4 oz grilled or baked salmon, flaked
    - Mixed greens
    - Cherry tomatoes, cucumber, and avocado slices
    - 1/2 cup plain Greek yogurt mixed with 1 scoop unflavored collagen powder, lemon juice, dill, and salt
    - Kale chips (baked or air-fried kale seasoned with olive oil and spices)
- Preparation:
    1. Toss greens with tomatoes, cucumber, and avocado. Top with flaked salmon.
    2. Drizzle with the collagen yogurt dressing. Garnish with crispy kale chips for a satisfying crunch.

9. Creamy Collagen Tomato Soup with Grilled Cheese Bites (Serves 2):

- Ingredients:
    - 1 tablespoon olive oil
    - 1 onion, chopped
    - 2 cloves garlic, minced
    - 1 (28-oz) can crushed tomatoes
    - 3 cups vegetable broth
    - 1 scoop beef or chicken collagen peptides
    - Fresh basil and oregano
    - Salt and pepper to taste
    - Whole wheat bread, cheese, and butter for grilled cheese bites
- Preparation:
    1. Sauté onion and garlic in olive oil until softened. Add tomatoes, broth, collagen peptides, herbs, and spices. Simmer for 15 minutes.
    2. Puree the soup if desired for a smoother texture. Serve with grilled cheese bites for a cozy and collagen-rich lunch.

10. Asian-Inspired Noodle Salad with Collagen-Marinated Shrimp and Peanut Sauce (Serves 2):

- Ingredients:
  - 1 cup cooked noodles (rice noodles, soba noodles, etc.)
  - 12 shrimp, marinated in 1 tablespoon rice vinegar, soy sauce, ginger, and 1 scoop fish collagen peptides
  - Shredded carrots, cucumber, bell peppers
  - Baby spinach
  - Asian-inspired peanut sauce (mix peanut butter, soy sauce, rice vinegar, lime juice, ginger, and sriracha)

Preparation:

1. Stir-fry or grill your marinated shrimp until cooked through.
2. Toss noodles with veggies, spinach, and shrimp. Drizzle with peanut sauce and enjoy a flavorful and collagen-rich Asian adventure

Dinnertime Delights

Hungry for a satisfying dinner but craving something healthy and bursting with flavor? Look no further! These 7 collagen-rich recipes are here to tantalize your taste buds and fuel your body with the protein it needs to thrive:

1. Collagen-Crusted Salmon with Roasted Brussels Sprouts and Lemon Butter (Serves 2):

- Ingredients:
    - 2 salmon fillets
    - 1/4 cup almond flour
    - 2 tablespoons parmesan cheese
    - 1 tablespoon chopped fresh herbs (dill, parsley, etc.)
    - 1 teaspoon paprika
    - 1/2 teaspoon salt and pepper
    - 1 cup Brussels sprouts, halved
    - Olive oil
    - Lemon butter (1 tablespoon butter softened with 1 teaspoon lemon juice)
    -
- Preparation:
1. Preheat oven to 400°F (200°C). Mix almond flour, parmesan cheese, herbs, paprika, salt, and pepper in a shallow dish.

2. Coat salmon fillets with the mixture, pressing gently to adhere. Arrange on a baking sheet lined with parchment paper.
3. Toss Brussels sprouts with olive oil and season with salt and pepper. Spread around the salmon.
4. Bake for 15-20 minutes, or until salmon is cooked through and Brussels sprouts are tender.
5. Drizzle with lemon butter before serving. Enjoy a flaky, flavorful, and collagen-rich masterpiece!

2. Beef Stir-Fry with Collagen Bone Broth and Veggies (Serves 4):

- Ingredients:
    - 1 tablespoon olive oil
    - 1 pound lean beef, thinly sliced
    - 1 cup chopped mixed vegetables (broccoli, carrots, bell peppers, etc.)
    - 1 cup collagen bone broth
    - 1 tablespoon soy sauce
    - 1 tablespoon rice vinegar
    - 1 teaspoon ginger paste
    - 1/2 teaspoon garlic powder

- Cornstarch slurry (1 tablespoon cornstarch mixed with 2 tablespoons water)
  - Chopped green onions and sesame seeds (optional)
- Preparation:
1. Heat olive oil in a large wok or skillet over medium-high heat. Stir-fry beef until browned.
2. Add vegetables and cook for 2-3 minutes, until slightly softened.
3. In a small bowl, whisk together collagen bone broth, soy sauce, rice vinegar, ginger paste, and garlic powder.
4. Pour the sauce into the wok and bring to a simmer. Thicken with cornstarch slurry if desired.
5. Garnish with chopped green onions and sesame seeds (optional) and serve over rice or noodles. A quick and easy collagen-powered stir-fry adventure!

3. Baked Chicken with Collagen Pesto and Creamy Mushrooms (Serves 4):

- Ingredients:
  - 4 boneless, skinless chicken breasts

- - 1/2 cup prepared pesto with 1 scoop of unflavored collagen powder mixed in
    - 1 tablespoon olive oil
    - 1/2 pound mushrooms, sliced
    - 1/2 cup heavy cream
    - 1/4 cup grated Parmesan cheese
    - Salt and pepper to taste
- Preparation:
1. Preheat oven to 375°F (190°C). Spread pesto evenly over chicken breasts.
2. Heat olive oil in a skillet over medium heat. Add mushrooms and cook until golden brown.
3. Stir in heavy cream, Parmesan cheese, salt, and pepper. Bring to a simmer and let thicken slightly.
4. Transfer the chicken to a baking dish and pour the mushroom sauce over the top.
5. Bake for 20-25 minutes, or until chicken is cooked through. Tender, juicy chicken infused with the delightful flavors of collagen pesto and creamy mushrooms – pure dinnertime bliss!

4. Collagen-Infused Slow Cooker Chili with Ground Turkey and Beans (Serves 4-6):

- Ingredients:
  - 1 tablespoon olive oil
  - 1 onion, chopped
  - 2 cloves garlic, minced
  - 1 pound ground turkey
  - 1 (28-oz) can diced tomatoes
  - 1 (15-oz) can of kidney beans, drained and rinsed
  - 1 (15-oz) can black beans, drained and rinsed
  - 1 cup beef or chicken collagen bone broth
  - 1 tablespoon chili powder
  - 1 teaspoon cumin
  - 1/2 teaspoon smoked paprika
  - Salt and pepper to taste
- Preparation:
1. Heat olive oil in a skillet over medium heat. Sauté onion until softened and slightly golden. Add garlic and cook for another minute until fragrant. Transfer to your slow cooker.
2. Brown the ground turkey in the same skillet, breaking it up with a spoon. Drain any excess fat and add the browned turkey to the slow cooker.
3. Stir in diced tomatoes, kidney beans, black beans, collagen bone broth, chili powder,

cumin, smoked paprika, salt, and pepper. Mix well to combine.

4. Cover and cook on low for 6-8 hours, or on high for 4-5 hours. Serve hot with your favorite chili toppings like shredded cheese, chopped onions, sour cream, and avocado. This slow-cooker chili simmers with rich collagen flavors, making it a hearty and satisfying way to end your day.

5. One-Pan Roasted Cod with Collagen, Tomatoes, and Herbs (Serves 4):

- Ingredients:
    1. 4 cod fillets
    2. 1 tablespoon olive oil
    3. 1/2 teaspoon salt and pepper
    4. 1 (14.5-oz) can diced tomatoes
    5. 1/2 red onion, sliced
    6. 1/2 cup kalamata olives, halved
    7. 1 cup cherry tomatoes, halved
    8. 1 tablespoon chopped fresh oregano
    9. 1 tablespoon chopped fresh parsley
    10. 1 scoop lemon collagen peptides
- Preparation:
1. Preheat oven to 400°F (200°C). Arrange cod fillets in a single layer on a large baking sheet lined with parchment paper. Drizzle

with olive oil and season with salt and pepper.

2. Stir together diced tomatoes, red onion, kalamata olives, cherry tomatoes, oregano, parsley, and collagen peptides in a bowl. Spoon the mixture around the cod fillets.

3. Bake for 15-20 minutes, or until cod is cooked through and tomato mixture is bubbly. A simple yet flavorful one-pan wonder, perfect for a busy weeknight!

6. Spicy Cajun Shrimp with Collagen Zucchini Noodles and Bell Peppers (Serves 2):

- Ingredients:
    1. 1 pound large shrimp, peeled and deveined
    2. 1 tablespoon olive oil
    3. 1 teaspoon Cajun seasoning
    4. 1/2 teaspoon salt and pepper
    5. 2 zucchini, spiralized into noodles
    6. 1 red bell pepper, sliced
    7. 1 yellow bell pepper, sliced
    8. 1/4 cup chicken broth
    9. 1 tablespoon chopped fresh parsley
- Preparation:

1. Heat olive oil in a large skillet over medium-high heat. Toss shrimp with Cajun seasoning, salt, and pepper. Add to the

skillet and cook for 2-3 minutes per side, until just pink and cooked through.

2. Add zucchini noodles, bell peppers, and chicken broth to the skillet. Stir-fry for 3-4 minutes until zucchini noodles are tender-crisp.

3. Garnish with chopped parsley and serve immediately. This quick and spicy dish packs a collagen punch with juicy shrimp and zucchini noodles – a flavorful and light dinner option.

7. Collagen-Enriched Coconut Curry Chickpea and Sweet Potato Stew (Serves 4):

- Ingredients:
    1. 1 tablespoon olive oil
    2. 1 onion, chopped
    3. 2 cloves garlic, minced
    4. 1 tablespoon curry powder
    5. 1 teaspoon ground ginger
    6. 1/2 teaspoon turmeric
    7. 1 (14.5-oz) can diced tomatoes
    8. 1 (15-oz) can coconut milk
    9. 1 cup vegetable broth
    10. 1 (15-oz) can chickpeas, drained and rinsed
    11. 1 sweet potato, peeled and diced
    12. 1 scoop unflavored collagen powder

13. Chopped cilantro and lime wedges (optional)

- Preparation:

1. Heat olive oil in a large pot or Dutch oven over medium heat. Sauté onion and garlic until softened. Add curry powder, ginger, and turmeric, and cook for another minute until fragrant.

2. Stir in diced tomatoes, coconut milk, vegetable broth, chickpeas, sweet potato, and collagen powder. Bring to a simmer and cook for 20-25 minutes, or until the sweet potato is tender.

3. Garnish with chopped cilantro and lime wedges (optional) and serve over rice or quinoa. This creamy and flavorful stew is packed with plant-based protein and a collagen boost, making it a nourishing and satisfying dinner choice.

Feel free to get creative and adjust these recipes to your preferences and dietary needs. The key is to embrace the versatility of collagen-rich ingredients and experiment with different flavors and textures to create delicious and nutritious meals that fuel your body.

Snacks and sides

Need a satisfying bite between meals but craving something healthy and collagen-packed? Look no further! These 5 delicious and easy-to-make snacks are bursting with flavor and nutrition to keep you energized all day long:

1. Collagen Bites: No-Bake Energy Balls with Nuts, Seeds, and Dried Fruit (Makes 15-20 balls):

- Ingredients:
  - 1/2 cup rolled oats
  - 1/4 cup chopped nuts (almonds, walnuts, pecans, etc.)
  - 1/4 cup chopped dried fruit (cranberries, apricots, raisins, etc.)
  - 1/4 cup sunflower seeds
  - 1/4 cup chia seeds
  - 1 tablespoon honey or maple syrup
  - 1 tablespoon nut butter (almond, peanut, etc.)
  - 1 scoop unflavored collagen powder
- Preparation:
1. Combine all ingredients in a bowl and mix well until everything sticks together.
2. Roll the mixture into bite-sized balls.
3. Refrigerate for at least 30 minutes for a firmer texture.

4. Pop one (or two!) in your mouth whenever you need a collagen-powered energy boost!

2. Homemade Collagen Granola with Nuts, Seeds, and Spices (Makes about 6 cups):

- Ingredients:
    - 3 cups rolled oats
    - 1/2 cup chopped nuts (almonds, pecans, hazelnuts, etc.)
    - 1/4 cup sunflower seeds
    - 1/4 cup pumpkin seeds
    - 1/4 cup coconut flakes
    - 1/4 teaspoon cinnamon
    - 1/4 teaspoon nutmeg
    - 1/4 teaspoon ground ginger
    - 1/8 teaspoon salt
    - 1/3 cup honey or maple syrup
    - 1 tablespoon olive oil
    - 1 scoop unflavored collagen powder

Preparation:

1. Preheat oven to 350°F (175°C). Line a baking sheet with parchment paper.
2. In a large bowl, combine oats, nuts, seeds, coconut flakes, spices, and salt.

3. In a separate bowl, whisk together honey or maple syrup, olive oil, and collagen powder.
4. Pour the wet ingredients over the dry ingredients and toss until evenly coated.
5. Spread the mixture evenly on the baking sheet.
6. Bake for 20-25 minutes, stirring once or twice during baking, until golden brown and crispy.
7. Let cool completely, then store in an airtight container for up to 2 weeks. Enjoy a crunchy and collagen-rich granola on yogurt, cereal, or even as a standalone snack

3. Collagen-Infused Hummus with Roasted Vegetables (Makes about 2 cups):

- Ingredients:
    - 1 (15-oz) can chickpeas, drained and rinsed
    - 1/4 cup tahini
    - 2 tablespoons olive oil
    - 2 tablespoons lemon juice
    - 1 clove garlic, minced
    - 1/2 teaspoon salt
    - 1/4 teaspoon cumin
    - 1 scoop unflavored collagen powder

- Roasted vegetables of your choice (sliced bell peppers, zucchini, broccoli, etc.)
- Preparation:

1. Preheat oven to 400°F (200°C). Toss your chosen vegetables with olive oil and salt, then roast for 20-25 minutes until tender and slightly browned.
2. In a food processor, combine chickpeas, tahini, olive oil, lemon juice, garlic, salt, cumin, and collagen powder. Blend until smooth and creamy.
3. Transfer the hummus to a serving bowl and top with roasted vegetables. Enjoy with pita bread, vegetables, or crackers for a protein-packed and collagen-rich snack.

4. Collagen Yogurt Parfait with Berries and Granola (Makes 1 serving):

- Ingredients:
    - 1 cup plain Greek yogurt
    - 1 scoop unflavored collagen powder
    - 1/2 cup fresh berries (blueberries, raspberries, strawberries, etc.)
    - 1/4 cup homemade collagen granola (from recipe above)

o Drizzle of honey or maple syrup
   (optional)

- Preparation:

1. In a bowl, mix together Greek yogurt and collagen powder until well combined.

2. Layer the yogurt in a parfait glass or bowl. Top with fresh berries and homemade collagen granola.

3. Drizzle with honey or maple syrup (optional) and enjoy a refreshing and delicious collagen-rich treat!

5. Crispy Baked Collagen Sweet Potato Fries with Spicy Mayo (Makes 2-3 servings):

- Ingredients:
  1. 2 large sweet potatoes, peeled and cut into thick fries
  2. 1 tablespoon olive oil
  3. 1/2 teaspoon paprika
  4. 1/4 teaspoon salt
  5. 1/4 teaspoon black pepper
  6. 1 scoop unflavored collagen powder
  7. For the Spicy Mayo:
     - 1/2 cup mayonnaise
     - 1 teaspoon Sriracha or hot sauce
     - 1/4 teaspoon cayenne pepper

- ■ Pinch of paprika
- Preparation:
    1. Preheat oven to 400°F (200°C). Line a baking sheet with parchment paper.
    2. In a large bowl, toss sweet potato fries with olive oil, paprika, salt, pepper, and collagen powder until evenly coated.
    3. Spread the fries in a single layer on the prepared baking sheet.
    4. Bake for 20-25 minutes, flipping halfway through cooking, until golden brown and crispy.
    5. While the fries are baking, combine mayonnaise, Sriracha or hot sauce, cayenne pepper, and paprika in a small bowl. Mix well.
    6. Serve the crispy sweet potato fries hot with the spicy mayo for a delightful and collagen-rich side dish or snack.

Feel free to experiment with different flavors and ingredients to customize these snacks to your taste. The key is to find healthy and tasty ways to incorporate collagen into your diet and keep your body fueled throughout the day. So grab your ingredients, get creative, and start snacking the collagen-rich way!

Bonus

Weekly Collagen Grocery List:

Feel free to adjust it based on your chosen recipes and dietary needs!

- Fresh Produce:
    - 1 head romaine lettuce
    - 1 bunch mixed greens
    - 1 avocado
    - 1 bunch broccoli
    - 1 bell pepper (red, yellow, or orange)
    - 1 cucumber
    - 1 cup cherry tomatoes
    - 1/2 cup blueberries
    - 1/2 cup raspberries
    - 1 sweet potato
    - 1 bunch bananas
- Proteins:
    - 1 pound salmon fillets
    - 1 pound boneless, skinless chicken breasts
    - 1 pound ground turkey
    - 1 can canned tuna
    - 1 can lentils
    - 1 can chickpeas
    - 1 container plain Greek yogurt

- Pantry Staples:
    - Whole wheat bread or tortillas
    - Brown rice or quinoa
    - Nuts and seeds (almonds, walnuts, sunflower seeds, chia seeds)
    - Olive oil
    - Lemon juice
    - Honey or maple syrup
    - Spices (paprika, cumin, chili powder, ginger, etc.)
    - Collagen peptides (unflavored or flavored)
- Bonus:
    - Spices for roasting vegetables (rosemary, thyme, garlic powder)
    - Fresh herbs (parsley, dill, cilantro)
    - A block of tofu or tempeh for vegetarian options

Create Your Own Collagen-Inspired Dishes!

Recipe:

Ingredients:

Instructions:

Create Your Own Collagen-Inspired Dishes!

Recipe:

Ingredients:

Instructions:

Create Your Own Collagen-Inspired Dishes!

Recipe:

Ingredients:

Instructions:

Create Your Own Collagen-Inspired Dishes!

Recipe:

Ingredients:

Instructions:

Create Your Own Collagen-Inspired Dishes!

Recipe:

Ingredients:

Instructions:

Create Your Own Collagen-Inspired Dishes!

Recipe:

Ingredients:

Instructions:

Create Your Own Collagen-Inspired Dishes!

Recipe:

Ingredients:

Instructions:

Create Your Own Collagen-Inspired Dishes!

Recipe:

Ingredients:

Instructions:

Create Your Own Collagen-Inspired Dishes!

Recipe:

Ingredients:

Instructions:

Create Your Own Collagen-Inspired Dishes!

Recipe:

57

Ingredients:

Instructions:

Create Your Own Collagen-Inspired Dishes!

Recipe:

Ingredients:

Instructions:

Create Your Own Collagen-Inspired Dishes!

Recipe:

Ingredients:

Instructions:

There are endless possibilities when it comes to adding collagen to your diet and creating delicious meals. Be a culinary explorer, experiment with flavors and textures, and most importantly, have fun!

Embrace the collagen revolution and cook up your own personal collage of flavor and nourishment.

Happy cooking